Primary Care Case Studies for Nurse Practitioners

Lydia Burke

Primary Care Case Studies for Nurse Practitioners
Lydia Burke

ISBN: 978-1-905539-23-9

First published 2008

British Library Catalogue in Publication Data
A catalogue record for this book is available from the British Library

Notice
Clinical practice and medical knowledge constantly evolve. Standard safety precautions must be followed, but, as knowledge is broadened by research, changes in practice, treatment and drug therapy may become necessary or appropriate. Readers must check the most current product information provided by the manufacturer of each drug to be administered and verify the dosages and correct administration, as well as contraindications. It is the responsibility of the practitioner, utilising the experience and knowledge of the patient, to determine dosages and the best treatment for each individual patient. Any brands mentioned in this book are as examples only and are not endorsed by the Publisher. Neither the publisher nor the authors assume any liability for any injury and/or damage to persons or property arising from this publication.

The Publisher

To contact M&K Publishing write to:
M&K Update Ltd · The Old Bakery · St. John's Street
Keswick · Cumbria CA12 5AS
Tel: 01768 773030 · Fax: 01768 781099
publishing@mkupdate.co.uk
www.mkupdate.co.uk

Designed and typeset by Mary Blood
Printed in England by Ferguson Print, Keswick

Primary Care Case Studies
for Nurse Practitioners

OTHER CLINICAL CARE BOOKS FROM M&K:

Routine Blood Results Explained 2/e
ISBN: 978-1-905539-38-3 · 2007

The Management of COPD in Primary and Secondary Care
ISBN: 978-1-905539-28-4 · 2007

Issues in Heart Failure Nursing
ISBN: 978-1-905539-00-0 · 2006

Arterial Blood Gas Analysis: an easy learning guide
ISBN: 978-1-905539-04-8 · 2008

Deep Vein Thrombosis and Pulmonary Embolism: a guide for practitioners
ISBN: 978-1-905539-51-2 · 2008

Self-assessment in Limb X-ray Interpretation
ISBN: 978-1-905539-13-0 · 2006

Self-assessment in Paediatric Musculoskeletal Trauma X-rays
ISBN: 978-1-905539-34-5 · 2008

Paediatric Minor Emergencies
ISBN: 978-1-905539-35-2 · 2008

Eye Emergencies: the practitioner's guide
ISBN: 978-1-905539-08-6 · 2008

The Clinician's Guide to Chronic Disease Management for Long Term Conditions: a cognitive-behavioural approach
ISBN: 978-1-905539-15-4 · 2008

Contents

Introduction

Primary Care is expanding because a wider range of health problems is now being managed outside of hospital settings. Practice nurses and nurse practitioners working alongside general practitioners in Primary Care settings are required to see and treat patients with a variety of minor and complex conditions. They therefore need skills in history-taking, physical assessment, diagnosing, prescribing and managing long-term conditions. Post-registration nurse students undertaking relevant programmes and modules need to be aware of the Nursing and Midwifery Council's regulatory framework for Advanced Nurse Practitioners (2005) and the Royal College of Nursing's Nurse Practitioner Competencies (2002). This book provides examples of patients that nurses who work in Primary Care may meet once they have achieved these competencies. The patient case-studies incorporate the variety that is usual in Primary Care. It is assumed that nurses who read this book will have experience in managing the care of babies, children, well young people, people for whom English is not their first language, people with mental health problems and older people with multiple health problems. Nurse practitioners should demonstrate sensitivity when working with people from different cultural groups and meet the related NMC competency (NMC 2005). Active learning and reflection is encouraged for each case study. It is expected that students will already have an understanding of the anatomy and physiology of the human body. They should have or be developing history-taking and physical assessment skills. Key texts for anatomy, physiology, pathophysi-ology, history-taking and physical assessment skills are included under Further Reading. In some of the case studies, students will be asked to describe their physical assessment of the patient. This will help reinforce the theoretical techniques of physical assessment. However expertise in physical assessment can only be acquired through supervised practice. Students should also be aware of the pathophysiology of common illnesses and health problems and their treatments.

These case studies are loosely based on interactions that the author has had with patients in Primary Care. The patients' names and situations are fictitious.

How to use this book

There are four chapters encompassing different types of problems typically seen in Primary Care. There are three or four case studies in each chapter. Several questions are embedded in the case studies to allow the reader to consider their knowledge and expertise relating to each case. Some questions encourage the reader to describe practical history taking and physical assessment activities for specific problems. Other questions will require the reader to look up information in texts or learning resources on the internet. These case studies can also be used by nurse lecturers to encourage groups of students to actively learn about managing illness in Primary Care. The answers are included at the end of each chapter. The reader should attempt to answer the questions as they occur in the text, rather than reading the answers at the end of the chapter. Once all the questions in one chapter have been attempted, then the reader can compare his or her answers with the answers at the end of the chapter. However it is acknowledged that students have different learning styles and some may benefit from looking up the answers immediately. These answers are the author's suggested good practice with inclusion of relevant, up-to-date references. They are not necessarily the only correct answers. For some questions, it is possible that the reader may put forward different answers that are equally valid and relevant to his or her clinical area.

Chapter One

Managing children and babies in primary care

Children, young people and babies make up a large component of the patients seen in Primary Care (Department of Health 2004). Children and babies are brought in to see nurses and health visitors for routine health screening, immunizations, feeding or sleep problems, minor trauma, allergies and infections. Children and babies are more susceptible to infections than adults as they have not yet acquired immunity. Parents and carers may bring them in with simple self-resolving viral illnesses because they need reassurance that the child does not have a serious infection such as meningitis. Assessing children can be challenging as they are often anxious, bored or uncooperative whilst in the surgery environment.

Nurse practitioners have the difficult role of diagnosing and managing minor health problems and teaching parents and carers how to manage these at home, whilst being vigilant for the rare serious problems. They should be up to date in child protection training, paediatric assessment and paediatric prescribing. They should also be aware of the average developmental progress for babies and children of different ages (Illingworth 1983).

Case Study A

Aisha

Soraya brings her daughter Aisha to the surgery because she has developed a rash. The receptionists book her into your walk-in clinic for advice and treatment. Before you call Aisha into your room, you check her electronic records. You see that she is two years old. She has been brought in to see you and your colleagues three times for minor upper respiratory infections and once for otitis media during the past year. She has had no serious illnesses and takes no regular medication. She is up to date with her childhood immunisations. The family's first language is English and they are of Asian origin. Soraya has also got her one-year-old son with her and four-year-old daughter. The two girls go to play with the toys in the corner. Soraya sits down holding her son. You observe that Aisha has built a tower of more than six bricks, has very good speech and is not wearing a nappy. She therefore appears to fulfil some of the developmental milestones for a two-and-a-half-year-old (Illingworth 1983). You use your communication skills to initiate the session.

A1. Describe your opening words and non-verbal communication:

Aisha's mother Soraya says: *'Its about Aisha – she's got a bad rash'*. She turns and calls her over. The little girl looks cheerful and there is no evidence of rash on her face or hands.

Soraya lifts up Aisha's dress.

'See her arms and tummy.'

Looking at her arms, you see hypo-pigmented skin at the left antecubital fossa and red, crusty, oozing lesions at the right antecubital fossa. There is localised redness surrounding the lesions. There is slight redness on the trunk and the skin feels very dry on palpation. You also check behind Aisha's legs and her back, but the skin appears normal there. She has a small, enlarged lymph node palpable in the right axilla. Her temperature is 36.4 degrees centigrade.

It is usual practice to structure the consultation so that history taking is carried out first and then the physical assessment is done. However, in short contingency appointments, it sometimes saves time to take a history and carry out examination simultaneously, which is what happens in this consultation.

A2. What further information do you need to help make a diagnosis?

A3. What is the significance of changes of pigmentation in pigmented skin?

A4. What findings suggest that Aisha has associated skin infection?

'When did you first notice the rash?' you ask.

'About a week ago'

'Is it anywhere else on her body?'

'Not that I've seen.'

'Is Aisha well at the moment?'

'Yes, well she's got a bit of a cold. She didn't go to school today.'

'Has she or anyone else in the family ever had eczema?'

'Eczema? Has she got eczema? She's never had eczema …'

'Umm, she could have, that's what it looks like… Do you know if this kind of dry skin condition runs in the family?'

'No-one's got skin problems, no.'

'Is Aisha allergic to anything that you know of?'

'No.'

'Does she suffer from asthma?'

'No.'

'Or anyone else in the family?'

'Well I used to have asthma when I was little, but I grew out of it.'

You are now at a stage in the consultation where it is time to make a provisional and differential diagnosis.

A5. Give a definition of atopic eczema and some differential diagnoses.

The one-year-old boy starts crying. Soraya asks:

'So what about the scabs on her arm here? Can I have some cream or something?'

You respond: 'Yes, and she will probably need some antibiotics by mouth for the infected skin on her right arm. She will need to have regular moisturising cream for the dry itchy skin that she has on her front and left arm. It looks as if she's got patches of eczema. The infection could have started from her scratching. If you use creams regularly, you can prevent it getting like this. Has Aisha ever been allergic to antibiotics?'

'No, she's had them before.'

'Is she allergic to penicillin?'

'No.'

A6. Suggest the appropriate treatment and a management plan. Describe a technique for measuring the correct amount of steroid cream to be applied.

You ask to see Aisha in one week to make sure that the localised flare-up of eczema is resolving.

A7. What information should you give when prescribing flucloxacillin?

When you see Aisha a week later, the infected crusts in her right antecubital fossa have disappeared. She still has dry lichenified skin and you encourage Soraya to use the emollients as frequently as possible. You remind her that the hydrous ointment and bath emollient are on repeat prescription so she should request more before they run out. You explain that eczema may not go away completely while Aisha is young, but the emollients will stop it worsening. Her skin is likely to improve as she gets older.

You print off some Patient Information Leaflets (PILs) from www.cks.library.nhs.uk and give them to Soraya to reinforce your advice:

1. Eczema – Atopic
2. Eczema – Emollients (Moisturisers)
3. Eczema – Fingertip Units for Topical Steroids

Case study B

Ben

You look at Ben's electronic records before calling his name, noting his age. He is five years old. You find that he has no significant past medical history, takes no medication and is up to date with his immunisations. His mother takes his hand and leads him down the corridor to your room. You greet his mother and him, observing his gait as he walks towards you. He is resisting his mother's encouraging hand, and therefore pulling back which makes it difficult to judge whether his steps are even. In the surgery, you invite Mrs Avrohom to sit down and tell you what the problem is. She says that she has noticed Ben limping for a few days. He walks to his primary school with his mother and older siblings each day. Over the past few days, he has been reluctant to put weight on his right leg, favouring his left leg. In the house, the limp was not as noticeable as he has been sitting playing or sitting being fed. His mother says that she can't remember any recent fall or accident. He is generally a cheerful active little boy who doesn't make a fuss when he hurts himself.

Having initiated the session and started taking a history from his mother, you now try to establish a rapport with Ben.

B1. What strategies do you adopt to help children feel at ease in the surgery?

B2. Write down three questions you would ask Ben's mother to help you make a provisional diagnosis.

1.

2.

3.

B3. Describe your physical assessment.

Physical assessment is essentially normal. You make a provisional diagnosis of musculoskeletal strain and encourage Mrs Avrohom to give Ben 7.5ml of ibuprofen after food three times daily whilst he has pain. You say that it is most likely a muscular problem but you will see him again in two days. Providing a follow-up appointment is safe practice, allowing the nurse to revise his or her provisional diagnosis if the illness does not follow the expected course. This contingency arrangement corresponds with Neighbour's 'safety netting' consultation checkpoint (1987) and the 'explanation/planning' component of the Calgary-Cambridge model (Kurtz & Silverman 1996).

When Ben is brought back, he is no better and still has a limp. Mrs Abrohom says that the ibuprofen does not make any difference to Ben's limp. You examine him again and he expresses discomfort on internally rotating his right hip. When you ask him where the pain is he points to his right knee and right femur. You are surprised that a five-year-old boy has limb or joint pain when there has been no apparent trauma. You decide to refer him to the paediatric team at the local hospital. The paediatrician organises an x-ray of his right knee and right hip. The right hip x-ray shows abnormalities suggestive of Perthes disease.

B4. Use your text books or on-line resources to find out about Perthes disease. Write a brief description of this condition.

Who does it affect most?

What are the symptoms?

What is the differential diagnosis?

Case Study C

Ellen

You are asked to see a three-month-old baby who has been coughing. Baby Ellen is carried in by her mother, 26-year-old Molly. You gain eye-contact, smile at mother and baby and introduce yourself as part of the 'connecting' process (Neighbour 1987).

C1. What questions do you ask to obtain a history?

C2. What examinations do you carry out?

Molly says that Ellen has been coughing for two days. She is still taking breast milk eagerly and has plenty of wet nappies. She has had a fever of 37.8 degrees centigrade, although today it has gone back to normal. She wakes once or twice in the night but this has not changed, and she is not excessively drowsy. From the history and examination you discuss the likely diagnosis of a viral respiratory infection that should resolve in a few days.

C3. What are the possible differential diagnoses?

You explain that Ellen has probably got a mild viral respiratory infection and her symptoms should gradually resolve over the next few days. You summarise the negative findings from the history and physical assessment. You put forward a management plan for Molly which involves observing Ellen, encouraging fluids and treating any pyrexia should it arise. This is part of Neighbour's 'Handing over' stage of the consultation (1987). In view of her young age, you give her a follow-up appointment in two days to review her respiratory symptoms again. When you see her again Ellen is coughing less, has no fever and is well. On examination there is no respiratory distress and her lungs are clear.

C4. What are the warning signs that should alert the mother to seek further advice?

Answers

Aisha

A1. Describe your non-verbal communication and opening words:

The Cambridge-Calgary Guide provides a structure for conducting the consultation starting with initiating the session (Silverman *et al.* 2005). Communication works best if you are sitting facing the person in an 'open' body position (not crossed arms and crossed legs) with good eye contact. Make sure your chair is the same height as your patient's (not higher). You may ask what seems to be the problem with Aisha in order to encourage the mother to tell you her concerns. Neighbour (1987) describes the initial introductions as 'connecting' which means establishing a rapport, focusing on intuitive hunches, taking a history and building up an impression from non-verbal and verbal communications.

A2. What further information do you need to help make a diagnosis?

You need to know the duration of the rash and whether it was triggered by something. You should find out if it is an itchy rash and ask if she is generally well at present. Ask if she has had a fever. You need to ask if Aisha's siblings or other household members have a similar rash. You should ask and check her records to see if she has a past history of skin problems or allergy. It is useful to find out if Soraya has been treating the rash with anything.

A3. What is the significance of changes of pigmentation in pigmented skin?

Inflammation, for example due to eczema or psoriasis, may cause changes in pigment and this happens more frequently in pigmented skin. Hypopigmentation is thought to be caused by inhibition of the melanocyte function if there is a rapid turnover of the epidermis. Hyperpigmentation can be caused by stimulation of melanocytes and/or retention of melanin granules in the dermis after there has been destruction of the basal layer of the epidermis. Inflammatory changes to pigmentation should resolve once the skin condition is treated and scratching ceases, although it may take weeks or months. (du Vivier 2002).

Answers

A4. What findings suggest that Aisha has infected eczema?

Findings that suggest Aisha has infected eczema are the yellow crusts and exudates, the local redness and the enlarged axillary lymph node.

A5. Give a definition of atopic eczema and some differential diagnoses.

Atopic eczema is a chronic, relapsing, inflammatory skin condition characterised by an itchy red rash that favours the skin creases (e.g. antecubital fossae and popliteal areas).

Skin infection (e.g. staphylococcal aureas impetigo)

Molluscum contagiosum

Infected insect bites

Scabies

A6. Suggest appropriate treatment and a management plan.

Flucloxacillin 250 mg/5ml syrup 5ml four times daily for seven days, to be taken 30 minutes before food (150 mls)

Hydrous ointment to be applied frequently (500 grams)

Hydrocortisone 1% to be applied sparingly twice a day for seven to fourteen days (15 grams).

Describe a technique for measuring the correct amount of steroid cream to be applied:

A fingertip unit of steroid cream or ointment is the amount squeezed onto the finger from the fingertip to the first crease. In an adult, this amount can treat an area of skin equivalent to twice the flat of the hand including the fingers. In a two-year-child like Aisha, a third of a fingertip unit will be enough to treat the same area.

A7. What information should you give when prescribing flucloxacillin?

Take an hour before food or on an empty stomach. Finish the prescribed course.

Ben

B1. What strategies do you adopt to help children feel at ease in the surgery?

'Connecting' with children in the primary care setting can be difficult (Neighbour 1987). It may be necessary to focus your attention on the parent or carer initially in order to avoid distressing the child. You can then offer the child a toy and look at this whilst indirectly making observations.

B2. What questions could you ask?

Is he still cheerful and active? Is he eating OK? Has he been sleeping in his usual pattern? Has he had a fever? Has he been given any analgesia, and has this made any difference to the leg pain?

B3. Describe your physical assessment.

Observe Ben standing – does he have a level pelvis? Observe his gait. Check for muscle wasting. Ask him to point to where it hurts.

Examine him on the couch to check internal and external rotation of the hips and knees using the roll test. The patient lies supine and the examiner rolls the hips into external and internal rotation. A positive test is when this movement invokes guarding or spasm, especially on internal rotation. Check flexion and extension of the hips and knees.

B4. Use your text books or on-line resources to find out about Perthes disease.

Write a brief description of this condition.

Perthes disease, also known as Legg-Calvé-Perthes (LCPD) disease or syndrome, is a childhood condition affecting the hip. Many theories have been proposed as to the cause, including trauma, infection, inflammation and congenital hip problems. It is currently thought that there is an interruption to the blood supply to the femoral epiphysis, physis or less commonly the metaphysis. When this happens, a part or all of the area involved temporarily dies and subchondral cortical bone infarction occurs. The acetabulum is not affected and articular cartilage continues to grow. Then revascularisation occurs and new bone ossification begins and some children revert to normal bone growth and development. However, a small percentage of children develop subchondral fracture and changes to the epiphyseal growth plate which causes pain.

Who does it affect most?

Most commonly Perthes disease is seen in the four to eight year age group, but it can occur in children aged two years up to teenagers. Boys tend to suffer more than girls by a ratio of four or five to one. LCPD can involve both hips in 10–12% of children, but does not occur simultaneously at exactly the same stage. LCPD has never been proven to be inherited although there are some studies that there can be an associated positive family history (www.perthes.org.uk).

What are the symptoms?

The symptoms of LCPD are varied. There may be intermittent mild hip or groin pain, which can be referred to the thigh or knee. The child may have an intermittent limp, sometimes worse on activity. On examination, there may be decreased internal rotation and/or abduction. There may be atrophy of the thigh muscles. The affected leg may be shorter than the other. The child may be shorter in height than children of the same age.

What is the differential diagnosis?

The differential diagnoses include tuberculosis, sickle cell anaemia, rheumatoid arthritis, pelvic fracture, hypothyroidism, septic hip, congenital dislocated hip, lymphoma and slipped femoral capital epiphysis (Jarvis 2004).

Ellen

C1. What questions do you ask to obtain a history?

What is the duration and frequency of Ellen's cough? Does she seem to struggle for breath? Has she had a fever? Does she have a runny nose? Is she feeding less? Do you breast or bottle feed? Does she seem more drowsy than normal? Does the cough disturb her sleep? Does she still have plenty of wet nappies? Is the parent concerned that there is something seriously wrong? Was Ellen born prematurely? Were there any problems during her birth or afterwards?

C2. What examinations do you carry out?

Check Ellen's weight and temperature. Detection of fever should be done with an electronic thermometer in the axilla, or a chemical dot thermometer in the axilla or an infra-red tympanic thermometer in the ear (NICE 2007). If the child has a fever you should assess her colour, activity, respiration and hydration. Inspect her skin, lips and tongue to exclude pallor or cyanosis. Observe the child's alertness and note her muscle tone. Note whether she is content and smiling or crying. If she is crying, is it her normal cry? Check her head to exclude a bulging fontanelle. Undress her to check her skin for any rashes. Feel for enlarged lymph nodes in the submandibular, occipital, pre- and post-auricular and cervical areas. Use an otoscope to check the ears and tympanic membranes. Look for mucus and/or nasal flaring in the nostrils. Use a torch to check the pharynx. Carry out respiratory examination: count the respiratory rate; observe for use of accessory muscles or intercostal recession.

C3. What are the possible differential diagnoses?

Differential diagnosis is pneumonia, inhalation of foreign body, allergy and whooping cough.

C4. What are the warning signs that should alert the mother to seek further advice?

If Ellen develops a fever again, feeds less or not at all, becomes inappropriately drowsy, develops a non-blanching rash, has a high-pitched cry or has less wet nappies she should seek further advice. If the cough persists or worsens after the follow-up appointment, Molly should make another appointment for assessment of Ellen. If the mother has any concerns with her young baby she can come back to the surgery and be seen again at any time. If she is worried when the surgery is closed she can ring the out-of-hours service for advice.

Chapter Two

Managing common problems

Viral upper respiratory tract infections, low back pain, acne and eczema, urinary tract infections, rashes, warts, cellulitis, diarrhoea, constipation and minor injuries are some of the common conditions for which patients consult the nurses in primary care (Johnson *et al*. 2005). For patients requesting 'same day' appointments for acute minor illness it has been found that nurse practitioners provide good patient satisfaction and equivalent care to their GP colleagues (Horrocks *et al*. 2002). Although the problem may seem common and straightforward there may be underlying psychological problems or hidden agendas that need addressing (e.g. domestic violence or alcohol problems). Primary care Advanced Nurse Practitioners should be able to diagnose, treat and refer some psychological problems such as anxiety, depression, insomnia and addictions. Patient Health Questionnaires (e.g. PHQ-9) can be useful to help the practitioner judge the severity of depression or anxiety (www.depression-primarycare.co.uk/images/PHQ-9.pdf).

Health education is important in empowering the patient to recognise conditions that are self-limiting and important signs of more serious illness for which they should seek help.

The consultations should be documented in the patient's notes, whether electronic or paper. The problem-orientated medical record (POMR) and 'SOAP' structure, first described by Lawrence Weed (1969) helps structure your records. SOAP (subjective, objective, analysis/assessment, plan) is better extended to SOAPIER (subjective, objective, analysis/assessment, plan, implementation, evaluation and review/revision) for use by nurse practitioners in Primary Care. The subjective and objective information often corresponds to the 'history of presenting complaint' part of the history-taking process (Silverman *et al.* 2005). The PQRST symptoms analysis tool provides a useful framework to structure your questions (Walsh 2005). This includes questions about provocative-palliative factors, quality, region, severity and temporal or timing characteristics of symptoms. this (Gonce Morton 1990).

Case Study D

Jon

According to the records Jon is a 35-year-old man who joined your practice six weeks ago. You look at his Primary Care records before you call him to your consulting room.

The notes are as follows:

Current problems

Chronic rhinitis.

Past medical history

Discoid eczema twenty years ago.

Assault – fracture to right fourth metacarpal bone.

Fracture of tibia and fibula ten years ago.

Childhood viral meningitis aged five years old, good recovery.

Current medication

Beclomethasone nasal spray. Two puffs twice a day. One spray. (Repeat prescription.)

Recent past medication

Amoxicillin capsules 500mg. Three times a day. 21 capsules.

Smoking history

He smokes 30 cigarettes a day.

Social history

Jon works as a freelance plasterer. He lives in a rented flat with his girlfriend. After you call Jon's name, he walks slowly to your consulting room leaning on a stick. He sits down carefully and starts speaking immediately. He says 'I've done my back in. It's really bad and I can't do my job, and can hardly get about. I've borrowed this stick to get here. I've been lying in bed but its not helping.' This will be written up as the 'subjective' element of record keeping. You need to gain more objective factual information.

D1. Write down ten questions you would ask that incorporate the 'PQRST' structure.

1.

2.

3.

4.

5.

6.

7.

8.

9.

10.

Jon tells you that his back pain flared up three days ago and is persisting. He has been working very hard on a job, lifting heavy bags of plaster and reaching over his head to plaster ceilings. He does not remember any sudden onset of pain. The pain came on slowly throughout the day until it was bad enough to stop him working. He managed to sleep OK but woke up with back pain. He describes his pain as '7 or 8' on a visual analogue scale of one to ten (Wewers & Lowe 1990). It does not radiate anywhere. He has no fever, no bladder or bowel problems and no numbness.

D2. Describe your physical assessment.

D3. What are the back pain 'red flag' criteria?

On examination, there is no cervical lordosis, thoracic kyphosis or lumbar lordosis. There is no tenderness of the cervical, thoracic, lumbar or sacral vertebrae. There is tenderness around the left sacro-iliac joint. He has restricted flexion of the lumbar spine, although he takes off and puts on his trousers with ease. When testing straight leg raising, you find that he can lift his left leg to 70 degrees and his right leg to 90 degrees. His patella tendon reflexes are intact. You carry out a brief neurological examination and find out that his sensation is intact to deep and light touch, heat and cold, and vibration. You make a diagnosis of acute mechanical musculo-skeletal back strain, likely to be associated with his work as a plasterer.

D4. What is the difference between mechanical low back pain and non-mechanical low back pain?

D5. What are the differential diagnoses?

D6. Jon asks if he can have an x-ray of his back – how do you respond?

After gathering 'subjective', 'objective' and 'analytical/assessment' information to record, it is now time to suggest and document the 'plan' (Weed 1969).

D7. Put forward a management plan for Jon.

Once the plan (P) has been implemented (I) it is appropriate to evaluate (E) the consultation. Such evaluation in record keeping ties in with Roger Neighbour's 'house-keeping' where the nurse must reflect on the effectiveness of the consultation, before embarking on the next (2004). The arrangements for reviewing (R) the patient are also documented in the notes. Jon is asked to come back in two weeks if his symptoms are not improving. He is given a patient information leaflet on low back pain: http://www.patient.co.uk/showdoc/23068686/.

Case Study E

Gulsen

Gulsen, who is 16 years old, comes to see you with her older sister. She is from a Turkish family but was born in the UK. Gulsen's sister explains the problem that will be documented in the 'subjective' part of the consultation. She says that Gulsen has been getting bad spots on her face and would like some treatment. Gulsen's friend has been put on the pill for her spots and now they have gone and she would also like to try the pill.

As you are listening you notice that Gulsen has a few closed comedones on her forehead and chin. There are no pustules and no scars on her face.

You need objective information.

E1. Write down five questions that you would ask.

1.

2.

3.

4.

5.

During the assessment stage of the consultation you carry out a clinical examination. On inspection, she has four or five closed comedones on her chin and two on her forehead. There are no pustules present. Her cheeks, neck, chest and back are free from acne. There is no scarring of her skin. She is of normal weight for her height and has no hirsutism. Her blood pressure is 110/68mmHg.

During the history-taking process you find out that Gulsen takes no medication. She has a boyfriend. They are not sexually active yet but would like to be. Gulsen has regular periods and had her menarche aged 12 years. Her parents do not know that she has a boyfriend, but her older sister does. Her boyfriend is 17 years old. He already has condoms from the Young Persons' Sexual Health service.

You make a provisional diagnosis of mild acne vulgaris. Gulsen would like treatment for this. There seems to be a 'hidden agenda' in this consultation (Neighbour 1987, Silverman *et al.* 2005). You establish that Gulsen would like treatment for her skin and also to commence on the combined oral contraceptive pill.

E2. Describe how you would classify mild, moderate and severe acne vulgaris.

E3. What first line treatment would you recommend for mild acne vulgaris?

E4. Is it legal for you to prescribe the contraceptive pill to Gulsen?

You discuss her acne vulgaris and give Gulsen a patient information leaflet about acne: **http://www.patient.co.uk/showdoc/23068674/**

You also provide information about prevention of sexually transmitted infections and pregnancy. You have negotiated with Gulsen, hopefully influenced her and presented advice according to the 'handing over' stage of the consultation (Neighbour 1987). A prescription is written and you invite her to a follow-up appointment as a safety-netting arrangement.

Tony

Tony attends for a walk-in appointment complaining that he has had earache for two days. The pain is in his left ear and kept him awake last night. The hearing in this ear is dulled. Yesterday he tried cleaning out his ear with a cotton bud and it was very painful, and he noticed pale thin exudate on the cotton bud. His general health is good. He has never suffered from ear problems before. In the past he has suffered from mild eczema on his arms, legs and neck. He is a non-smoker. He drinks alcohol in moderation, approximately 16 units spread throughout the week. He enjoys swimming twice a week early in the morning before going to work as a physiotherapist. He is Caucasian. He lives with his girlfriend and two children.

F1. Describe your assessment of this man, including the correct way to hold an otoscope:

On examination you see that the outer third of the left auditory canal is scaly and inflamed. Using the otoscope you can see that the deeper auditory canal is red and swollen and there is pus-like exudate in the canal. The tympanic membrane is partially visible and appears normal. The right ear has a small amount of wax in the outer third of the auditory ear canal. The right tympanic membrane is clearly visible and the usual landmarks are seen. There are no enlarged lymph nodes palpable and his temperature is normal. His throat, mouth, teeth, gums and nose appear normal.

F2. What are the usual landmarks seen in a normal tympanic membrane?

F3. What is the difference between otitis media and otitis externa?

F4. Explain how otitis externa could lead to dulled hearing.

F5. What would you prescribe for otitis externa?

Tony is concerned about the wax in his right ear. He requests ear syringing.

F6. What are the contra-indications to ear irrigation?

You explain to Tony the diagnosis of otitis externa and write a prescription to treat this. You discuss the association between eczema and otitis externa and advise him to use regular emollients for his skin. You also explain that acute otitis externa is five times more common in swimmers as compared with non-swimmers (Raza *et al.* 1995). He needs to keep his ears dry so should use ear plugs in the water and avoid showering water in his ears. You explain that the ears are self-cleaning structures and that the use of cotton buds to clean out wax is unnecessary and can be harmful. You provide Tony with a public information leaflet on otitis externa:

http://www.patient.co.uk/showdoc/23068864/

Tony is given a follow-up appointment for one week's time to assess the response to treatment.

Answers

Jon

D1. Write down ten questions you would ask that incorporate the 'PQRST' structure.

Palliation/provocative questions:

You should ask if there have been any trigger factors to cause the back pain.

Has he taken any pain-relief and has this helped?

Are there any relieving or exacerbating factors?

Quality questions:

Where exactly is the pain?

Is the pain in one side or both sides of his back?

Is there any associated numbness or altered sensation (such as pins and needles)?

Severity questions:

On a visual analogue scale of 1–10, with 10 being the most severe pain imaginable and 0 being no pain, what number is the pain now? (Wewers & Lowe 1990).

Timing questions:

When did the pain start?

Does the pain radiate into the buttock or down the leg?

Is the pain persistent, or does it come and go?

Is the pain worse at night? Is the pain keeping him awake at night?

Other general questions:

How much alcohol is he drinking each day?

Is he using any street drugs?

Apart from the back pain, is he well at the moment? Any fever?

Is he experiencing any urinary symptoms?

Is there any problem with his bowels?

Is he currently depressed, anxious or feeling stressed?

D2. Describe your physical assessment.

Get permission to examine Jon. Explain that you need him to undress down to his underpants. Observe his gait, check for unsteadiness especially when turning. Inspect the back for scoliosis (unequal skin creases), cervical lordosis, thoracic kyphosis or lumbar lordosis. Observe his posture. Ask the patient to flex, extend and laterally flex his neck to check the cervical spine. To check the thoracic spine you should ask Jon to sit to eliminate rotation from his pelvis or legs. Ask him to rotate his thoracic spine.

To assess the lumbar spine he should then stand up. You can assess lumbar spine flexion by identifying two adjacent spinous processes, e.g. L4 and L5, and ask him to bend forwards. If the lumbar spine is flexing you should be able to feel the two processes separate slightly (www.jointzone.org.uk). Ask him to flex laterally at the lumbar spine.

Ask Jon to lie supine on the couch to test straight leg raising right and left. It is normal for both legs to reach 80–90° of flexion. Restriction of movement occurs if there is spinal or hip disease. If there is a nerve root problem at L4 or below raising the leg induces pain which increases if the foot is then dorsiflexed (Epstein *et al.* 2003).

D3. What are the back pain 'red flag' criteria?

There are several red flag criteria that call for urgent or immediate referral to an orthopaedic surgeon (NICE 2001):

● saddle anaesthesia (ask if the patient has noticed any numbness or strange sensations around the buttocks or between the legs)

● urinary problems, such as incontinence

● bowel problems – constipation, faecal incontinence

● change in sexual function – loss of feeling in the genitals.

Patients under the age of 20 years or over the age of 55 years are more likely to have a serious cause for their back pain. You should also be more prepared to refer the patient if there is a history of back injury, or non-mechanical progressive pain, or thoracic pain and/or widespread neurological symptoms. If they have had a past history of cancer, back pain could indicate metastases (www.cks.library.nhs.uk/back_pain_lower).

Answers

D4. What is the difference between mechanical low back pain and non-mechanical low back pain?

Mechanical low back pain is worse with physical activity, can be precipitated by lifting or bending, can be recurrent and often affects people aged 20–55 years. The pain is limited to the back or upper leg. The patient is systemically well and there is no evidence of nerve root distribution. 90% of people with mechanical low back pain are better within 6 weeks (Haslett *et al.* 2002). By contrast, non-mechanical pain is present all the time and does not usually vary. It is not made worse by activity. It may be caused by serious spinal pathology or gastric, pancreatic, colonic, prostatic or, in women, uterine/ovarian malignancies.

D5. What are the differential diagnoses?

Herniated intervertebral disc, vertebral fracture, osteoarthritis of apophyseal facet joints, ankylosing spondylosis, spinal tumour, metastases from an undiagnosed primary cancer.

D6. Jon asks if he can have an x-ray of his back – how do you respond?

You should explain that plain radiographs are not needed to confirm the diagnosis of acute mechanical low back pain and would be considered an unnecessary exposure to radiation. In young patients with persistent back pain x-ray may be useful to exclude ankylosing spondylosis. By the age of 50, 60% of women and 80% of men have radiographic features of spondylosis, with no correlation to the extent of the degeneration and the degree of back pain (Haslett *et al.* 2002).

D7. Put forward a management plan for Jon.

It is good advice to recommend that patients with back pain return to their usual activities as soon as possible. It was found that for acute or recurrent low back pain with or without referred leg pain, bed rest for 2–7 days was worse than placebo or ordinary activity (Waddell *et al.* 1996). Regular analgesia, such as paracetamol, and non-steroidal anti-inflammatory drugs (NSAIDs), such as ibuprofen may be helpful to relieve pain and improve mobility. You could also suggest that Jon try local heat or cold treatments, for example using alternate hot and cold water in the shower.

Jon may wish to seek out complementary therapies to help reduce his pain, such as acupuncture (www.backcare.org.uk).

You may wish to refer Jon to your local physiotherapy back pain service, or alternatively an osteopathy or chiropractor service if available.

You may also promote your surgery's smoking cessation services in case he ever wishes to try to quit smoking.

Gulsen

E1. Write down five questions you would ask.

Your questions need to focus on two issues – her skin problem and her request for the contraceptive pill:

When did the spots first appear?

How concerned are you about these spots?

Have you tried any medication for your skin?

Warn the patient that you also need to ask more personal questions about the need for the combined oral contraceptive pill – e.g. are you currently in a relationship?

Have you started having sex?

Do you need information about contraception and preventing sexually transmitted diseases?

Are your parents aware that you would like to commence the oral contraceptive pill?

E2. Describe how you would classify mild, moderate and severe acne vulgaris.

Mild acne is diagnosed when the patient has open and closed comedones with or without sparse inflammatory lesions.

Moderate acne describes numerous papules and pustules and more widespread non-inflammatory lesions.

Severe acne is diagnosed when the patient has extensive inflammatory lesions. There may also be nodules, pitting and scarring

(http://www.cks.library.nhs.uk/Acne_vulgaris/In_depth/References).

E3. What first line treatment would you recommend for mild acne vulgaris?

Benxoyl peroxide aquagel 2.5% – 10% for mild acne vulgaris once or twice daily.

E4. Is it legal for you to prescribe the contraceptive pill to Gulsen?

Yes, it is legal to prescribe the contraceptive pill. The Fraser Guideline criteria provide guidance in prescribing combined oral contraceptives to women aged less than 16 years who have not gained parental consent (Department of Health 2001).

It is also important to consider child protection issues in all patients under the age of 18 years, for example ensuring that sexual intercourse is consensual (Faculty of Family Planning and Reproductive Health Care Clinical Effectiveness Unit 2003)

Tony

F1. Describe your assessment of this man including the correct way to hold an otoscope:

Start by inspecting the face and pinnae for asymmetry or redness. Check Tony's temperature. Palpate the lymph nodes of the neck and throat: posterior and anterior auricular, occipital, submaxillary, submental, and the anterior and posterior cervical chain. Now focus on the good ear, the right ear. Inspect the pinna, outer meatus and adjacent scalp with a good light source. You may be able to see discharge, exudate, redness or swelling in the outer part of the auditory canal with the naked eye. Move the hair away if necessary. Check for previous surgery incision scars, discharge and signs of skin lesions. Gently palpate the mastoid area and move the pinna. Inspect the affected left ear in the same way. It is likely to be painful when you gently move the pinna in otitis externa.

Get your otoscope ready with a disposable speculum. Gently pull the pinna upwards and downwards to straighten the auditory canal. When inspecting a child's ear it is necessary to pull the pinna down and backwards to straighten their auditory canal. Hold the otoscope like a pen and put your little finger against the patient's head so that you get warning if they move their head. Use the light to check the ear canal and tympanic membrane. Adjust the direction of the otoscope to visualise all of the tympanic membrane. You should hold the otoscope in the left hand whilst inspecting the left ear and vice versa (www.entnursing.com, www.earcarecentre.com).

F2. What are the usual landmarks seen in a normal tympanic membrane?

The light reflex (at approximately 5 o'clock in the right ear, 7 o'clock in the left ear), handle of malleus, pars flaccida, pars tensa and anterior recess.

F3. What is the difference between otitis media and otitis externa?

Otitis media is inflammation of the middle ear. It can be acute with severe earache often preceded by upper respiratory tract infection. It is common in children (SIGN 2003). Otitis media can be chronic with effusion (glue ear). The cause of acute otitis media may be viral or bacterial.

Otitis externa is different because it affects the external ear, which includes inflammation of the auricle, the external ear canal or outer surface of the tympanic membrane. It can be localised (e.g. a furuncle) or diffuse. Otitis externa can be acute or become chronic. It may be caused by bacterial and fungal infections (e.g.staphylococci, streptococcoi, pseudomonas, candida or aspergillus), or allergic or irritant contact dermatitis.

F4. Explain how otitis externa could lead to dulled hearing.

Inflammation of the external ear canal often leads to temporary conductive hearing loss. Soundwaves which normally travel down the external ear canal freely to bounce against the tympanic membrane are obstructed by the narrowed canal and discharge. Otitis externa can also affect the outer surface of the tympanic membrane which impedes the conduction of soundwaves across the membrane to the malleus beneath.

F5. What would you prescribe for otitis externa?

Topical ear preparations are the first-choice treatment for acute otitis externa. Oral antibiotics are not usually necessary. Combined steroid and antibacterial and antifungal preparations such as Flumetasone and clioquinol ear drops (Locorten-Vioform) or astringent/acidic ear preparations, such as, acetic acid 2% (EarCalm) ear drops are cost-effective treatment for acute otitis externa

Answers

(http://www.cks.library.nhs.uk/otitis_externa). However there should be local joint formulary recommendations for your practice area.

F6. What are the contra-indications to ear irrigation?

- the patient has previously experienced complications following this procedure in the past

- there is a history of a middle ear infection in the last six weeks

- the patient has undergone ANY form of ear surgery (apart from grommets that have extruded at least 18 months previously and the patient has been discharged from the ENT Department)

- the patient has a perforation or there is a history of a mucous discharge in the last year

- the patient has a cleft palate (repaired or not)

- there is evidence of acute otitis externa with pain and tenderness of the pinna (www.earcarecentre.com).

Chapter Three

Assessing for serious or potentially life-threatening conditions

Most patients who come to seek treatment and advice from nurse practitioners do not have life-threatening conditions. If they are suffering from very serious illness or trauma they are more likely to attend an Emergency Department. However there are a few conditions that do not cause too much concern to the patient (or the patient's carer), but can develop into serious illness or have severe complications. There can be an atypical presentation of myocardial infarction for example (Brindle *et al*. 2003). The benefit of structured patient-centred history taking and expert, appropriate physical assessment usually helps to exclude serious life-threatening conditions, in addition to forming provisional diagnoses. Nurse practitioners should be confident to refer a patient for urgent in-patient assessment if they suspect a serious illness that cannot be treated in Primary Care. Nurses should not be hesitant in discussing the patient with a Primary Care or hospital colleague if they are unsure what action to take.

When critical incidents do occur, as inevitably they will, Primary Care teams should have clinical meetings to discuss what happened and devise strategies to ensure similar future incidents are prevented (van Zwanenburg & Harrison 2004).

Case Study G

Ahmed

Ahmed attends your walk-in clinic having told the receptionist that he has 'stomach pain'. He walks in slowly, slightly bent forward. He sits down carefully, guarding his abdomen with his arm and hand. He appears uncomfortable. You take a history and elicit that the abdominal pain started gradually three days ago.

G1. Write down nine questions, incorporating the PQRST analysis, that could help you make a diagnosis:

1.

2.

3.

4.

5.

6.

7.

8.

9.

You discover that when the pain started Ahmed says it was 'in the middle of the stomach' but now it has moved to his right lower side. He has had the pain since yesterday morning. He has not vomited and has no diarrhoea or constipation. He says the pain comes and goes. He does not feel unwell.

G2. List the nine anatomical segments of the anterior abdominal wall:

1.

2.

3.

4.

5.

6.

7.

8.

9.

G3. If Ahmed has appendicitis, what would you expect to find on examination?

After examination, you decide that it is likely Ahmed is suffering from appendicitis. You telephone the local hospital and ask to speak to the Surgical Registrar or SHO on call. They take the patient's details and ask him to come to the Emergency Department with a letter, where they will meet him. Ten days later Ahmed comes to see you again for suture removal following appendicectomy. You remove six sutures from his wound in the right iliac fossa ten days post-operatively and the wound is well healed. Two weeks later you receive a discharge summary confirming that Ahmed has had an appendicectomy. Post-operatively he does very well and is discharged after three days.

G4. Why do some cases of appendicitis get missed? What could be the consequence of missing the diagnosis of appendicitis?

G5. List some differential diagnoses of abdominal pain:

Case Study H

Maria

Maria comes to see you saying that her period was late and she is worried that she is pregnant. Her last menstrual period was five weeks ago and she normally has a period every 30 days. She has a boyfriend whom she has been seeing for the past two years. Maria has a three-year-old son from a previous relationship and she is not planning to have any more children. Her boyfriend usually uses condoms although there may have been an incident in the past month when the condom slipped off. Her past medical history includes Chlamydia infection five years ago, which was treated at the Sexual Health Clinic. She had a normal vaginal delivery at term when her son was born three years ago. Maria has had one suction termination of pregnancy operation ten years ago.

Pregnancy test is positive.

Maria is very unhappy and asks if you can arrange a termination for her.

You refer her to Women's Out-patients and write a letter. She is given an appointment for three weeks' time. Two days before her appointment, Maria comes to see you again as she has been bleeding on and off for the past week. The blood is dark red, sometimes almost black and of a thick consistency. She has no pain in her abdomen. You examine her.

On examination, there is some blood present at the cervical os. There is no pain on palpation of the pelvis. Maria feels well. She asks if she is having a miscarriage. This seems to be the most likely diagnosis but you say there is also the risk of the bleeding being caused by an ectopic pregnancy. You explain that her past history of Chlamydia infection is a risk factor for ectopic pregnancy. You arrange for her to be seen the next day in the local Early Pregnancy Assessment Unit, and advise her to attend A&E if she develops any pain or heavy bleeding. Unfortunately in the evening, Maria experiences sudden onset of severe pelvic pain and heavy vaginal bleeding. She feels faint and then collapses. Her boyfriend calls an ambulance and she is taken straight to surgery on arrival at the local hospital. Ruptured ectopic pregnancy is diagnosed. After surgical removal of the fallopian tube and three blood transfusions Maria stabilises and is admitted to a ward for observation.

H1. At what stage of the pregnancy does a tubal ectopic pregnancy usually cause symptoms?

H2. Is the number of ectopic pregnancies rising or falling?

H3. What are the factors that increase women's risk of ectopic pregnancy?

Case Study J

Ricardo Ortego

Ricardo does not speak English so he comes to see you with his sister. She says that he has a very sore throat and feels very tired. On closer questioning, you find out that the sore throat started approximately 24 hours ago. He has pain on swallowing, and he does not have a cough. He has not taken any tablets for pain. On examination, Ricardo's temperature is 38 degrees centigrade and he has tender enlarged anterior cervical lymph nodes on the left side. He has an enlarged red left tonsil partially covered in white exudate. The right tonsil is also red but not so enlarged. He is breathing and swallowing normally throughout the consultation.

You do not have any access to Ricardo's past medical history as he has just registered with your practice and he previously lived in Brazil. Ricardo's sister says that Ricardo has not had serious medical conditions before and has never been allergic to antibiotics.

J1. What are the provisional and differential diagnoses?

J2. What factors increase the possibility that the infection is bacterial in origin?

You make a diagnosis of tonsillitis and prescribe penicillin V 500mg twice daily for seven days. You ask him to buy paracetamol and ibuprofen from the pharmacist for the pain and fever. You ask him to come back if he is not improving. The next day Ricardo consults with your GP colleague. His throat does not feel any better and he has difficulty swallowing. Your colleague examines him and notices that his left tonsil is now much more swollen. He diagnoses left peritonsillar abscess. He speaks to the ENT surgical registrar on call and arranges for him to be seen via A&E. Ricardo is admitted for IV antibiotics and makes a full recovery.

J3. What could be the consequences of delaying treatment of peritonsillar abscess?

Case Study F

Helena

Helena comes to see you having requested an urgent appointment. The history of the presenting complaint is that she has woken up this morning with a high temperature and pain on urinating. She also has abdominal pain and backache. She has suffered from uncomplicated lower urinary tract infections on numerous occasions for the past two years. She often does not come to the surgery for antibiotics but takes over the counter remedies which help. Helena says that her symptoms are much worse than when she previously has had a urinary tract infection. You now need to gather objective information.

K1. What further questions should you ask Helena?

K2. What physical assessment and investigations do you recommend?

K3. What is the difference between a lower and an upper urinary tract infection?

K4. What is the usual treatment for an uncomplicated lower urinary tract infection confirmed on dipstick or microscopy, culture and sensitivity?

K5. What is the treatment for pyelonephritis?

K6. Describe your health education advice for women experiencing frequent urinary tract infections.

Having carried out physical assessment and tested her urine you make a provisional diagnosis of pyelonephritis. You contact the Medical Registrar on call and she agrees to assess her via the Emergency Department. You write a prescription for some broad-spectrum antibiotics.

You review Helena two weeks after her episode of pyelonephritis. She is now well. You discuss her past history of recurrent urinary tract infections and give her a leaflet on recurrent cystitis in women:
http://www.patient.co.uk/showdoc/23068975/

Answers

Ahmed

G1. Write down nine questions, incorporating the PQRST analysis, that could help you make a diagnosis:

1. When did the pain start (Timing)?

2. Is it constant or intermittent (Timing)?

3. Where exactly is the pain and has it moved anywhere (Radiation)?

4. Does anything make the pain better or worse (Provocative/Palliative)?

5. Is the pain affected by eating or having your bowels open (Provocative/Palliative)?

6. Have you had any nausea or vomiting with the pain?

7. Have you had a change in bowel habit?

8. Have you lost weight recently?

9. Have you been taking any medicines recently?

G2. List the nine anatomical segments of the anterior abdominal wall:

1. Right hypochondrium

2. Epigastrium

3. Left hypochondrium

4. Right lumbar region

5. Umbilical region

6. Left lumbar region

7. Right inguinal region

8. Suprapubic region

9. Left inguinal region

G3. If Ahmed has appendicitis, what would you expect to find on examination?

He will have pain in the right iliac fossa with possible rebound tenderness. He may have pyrexia. Digital rectal examination to the right will be very painful.

G4. Why do some cases of appendicitis get missed? What could be the consequence of missing the diagnosis of appendicitis?

The symptoms of appendicitis can be confused with viral gastroenteritis, food poisoning or irritable bowel syndrome. The consequence of missing the diagnosis of appendicitis and therefore delaying surgery can be ruptured appendix and peritonitis.

G5. List some differential diagnoses of abdominal pain:

Appendicitis, cholecystitis, gastroenteritis, irritable bowel syndrome, biliary colic, duodenal ulcer, hiatus hernia, dyspepsia, gastro-oesophageal reflux disease, stress-related symptoms.

Maria

H1. At what stage of the pregnancy does a tubal ectopic pregnancy cause symptoms?

Tubal ectopic pregnancies commonly cause symptoms in the sixth to seventh week of the pregnancy, but can be anytime between the fourth and the sixteenth week of pregnancy.

H2. Is the number of ectopic pregnancies rising or falling?

The number of ectopic pregnancies is rising. This is likely to be caused by the increase in pelvic inflammatory disease and sexually transmitted infections, such as Chlamydia.

H3. What are the factors that increase women's risk of ectopic pregnancy?

Factors that increase the risk of ectopic pregnancy are previous Chlamydia infection, previous pelvic inflammatory disease and previous tubal damage or surgery. Another risk factor is having assisted conception or in-vitro fertilisation. Use of the intrauterine contraception device and progesterone only pill are also associated with ectopic pregnancy as they prevent uterine pregnancy but do not prevent tubal pregnancy.

Ricardo

J1. What are the provisional and differential diagnoses?

The most likely diagnosis is acute viral tonsillitis or group A beta-haemolytic streptococcal tonsillitis. The differential diagnoses are viral pharyngitis, laryngitis, parainfluenza, influenza, Epstein–Barr virus, or peritonsillar abscess.

J2. What factors increase the possibility that the infection is bacterial in origin?

The majority of sore throats are viral in origin and will resolve spontaneously. Group A beta-haemolytic streptococcus is cultured in only 5–17% of adults with sore throat (Linder & Stafford 2001).

Centor's algorithm of clinical features (Centor *et al.* 1981) helps identify the significant features of streptococcal infection: 1. presence of tonsillar exudates, 2. tender anterior cervical lymphadenopathy, 3. the absence of cough and 4. a history of fever. In this case, Ricardo had all four of these clinical signs.

J3. What could be the consequences of delaying treatment of peritonsillar abscess?

Delaying treatment could lead to obstruction of the airway, brain damage or death.

Helena

K1. What further questions should you ask Helena?

You need to establish whether this is another lower urinary tract infection or a more serious upper urinary tract infection. You also need to exclude a sexually transmitted infection:

Are you suffering from nausea or vomiting?

Have you noticed any blood in your urine?

Does the back pain get worse when you pass urine?

Do you have any vaginal discharge?

Have you recently got together with a new partner?

Do you practice safe sex?

Have you ever suffered from sexually transmitted infections?

Did you suffer from urinary tract infections when you were a child?

Is there any chance that you are currently pregnant?

K2. What physical assessment and investigations do you recommend?

You should take Helena's temperature and pulse.

You should gently palpate Helena's abdomen and flanks.

You should dipstick a urine sample and also send one off for microscopy, culture and sensitivity.

K3. What is the difference between a lower and an upper urinary tract infection?

Lower urinary tract infection is the presence of pathogenic micro-organisms in the urine, urethra and bladder. Upper urinary tract infection (or pyelonephritis) is an infection of the kidney and renal pelvis. Upper urinary tract infection usually has more severe symptoms that develop more rapidly than lower urinary tract infection. The patient may have a high fever >39 degrees centigrade and unilateral flank pain. They may also have nausea, vomiting and diarrhoea. On palpation of the abdomen there is tenderness on deep palpation with upper urinary tract infection.

K4. What is the usual treatment for an uncomplicated lower urinary tract infection confirmed on dipstick or microscopy, culture and sensitivity?

You should check your local prescribing guidelines. Usually Trimethoprim 200mg twice a day for three days is recommended, unless the patient has had an adverse reaction to Trimethoprim in the past.

K5. What is the treatment for pyelonephritis?

Oral antibiotics should be commenced immediately according to local policy and the British National Formulary (2007). If the patient has fever and other systemic symptoms they should be referred to hospital straight away. If the patient does not respond to oral antibiotics within 48 hours they should be referred to hospital. They should also be referred if they are pregnant, have severe nausea and vomiting, have diabetes, have functional or structural urinary tract abnormalities (http://www.cks.library.nhs.uk/Pyelonephritis_acute).

K6. Describe your health education advice for women experiencing frequent urinary tract infections.

If possible patients should pass urine before and after sex. They should try to avoid getting dehydrated by drinking fluids regularly. There is conflicting research on whether patients should drink excess fluids – increased fluid intake increases the urinary flow which may cause increased discomfort. There is also limited evidence to support the benefits of cranberry juice. (www.cks.library.nhs.uk/search/0/urinary_tract_infection).

Patients with vaginal irritation should avoid washing with soap. They should be instructed to use toilet tissue from front to back after using the toilet to prevent contamination by faecal bacteria.

Antibiotic prophylaxis should be considered if the patient has more than three urinary tract infections in one year – either post-coital if UTI is related to sex or for three months if unrelated to sex.

Chapter Four

Managing Patients with Multiple Health Problems

With the increasing ageing population and more treatments for illness (Bowling 2005), it is not surprising that an increasing group of patients consult with multiple health problems. Some conditions, such as diabetes mellitus, will be managed in longer annual review appointments. However now and then patients will consult with nurse practitioners for two or three problems within a ten minute appointment slot. It is very difficult to address the problems effectively in such a short time. In addition, having multiple health problems usually means that the patient will be taking several different medications. This can lead to drug interactions, side-effects and poor concordance (Royal Pharmaceutical Society of Great Britain 1997).

When patients have multiple health problems, nurse practitioners need to prioritise the more urgent problems and assess and treat these in the time available. They should provide follow-up appointments to deal with further problems. They should be able to carry out review of medication to prevent drug interactions and improve concordance.

Case Study L

James

James is a 73-year-old man who comes to see you with two problems. He has had pain in his left ankle on and off over the past year. He has been taking ibuprofen tablets every day but they give him heartburn. He now says that he has had pain in his chest for the past two days.

You note from his records that he was diagnosed with essential hypertension nine years ago. He takes Amlodipine 10mg every day. He is an ex-smoker and stopped smoking twenty years ago. James now lives alone, having separated from his wife fifteen years ago. He has had minor acute problems of upper respiratory tract infection, wax in his ear and back ache during the past ten years. He has a family history of stroke, diabetes and hypertension. He has no family history of ischaemic heart disease.

L1. Write down six questions you should ask related to his chest pain:

1.

2.

3.

4.

5.

6.

L2. Write down three questions you would ask related to his ankle pain:

1.

2.

3.

You find out that James has intermittent chest pain that he describes as 7/10 on a pain score. He says that the pain is worse after meals and worse after taking ibuprofen. Sometimes the pain is also in his upper abdomen. He has no associated diarrhoea or constipation.The chest pain becomes worse during walking or going up stairs.

James says that his left ankle aches even when he is resting. Sometimes the ankle swells up and he has burning pain on weight-bearing which restricts his ability to go shopping. He has not noticed any redness of the ankle joint.

L3. Describe your physical examination of the cardiovascular system:

L4. Describe your examination of his ankles:

After you have examined his cardiovascular system you document the following: No JACCOLD (jaundice, anaemia, cyanosis, clubbing, oedema, lymphadenopathy or dehydration). BP 138/82mmHg. Pulse 86 regular. Left and right tibial and pedal pulses – weak. JVP not raised, no evidence of mediastinal shift or ventricular hypertrophy. HS 1+2 + 0. No heaves or thrills on palpation. Lungs clear, no respiratory distress, respiratory rate is 24 breaths per minute.

On examination of his left ankle, there is swelling medially and laterally below the malleoli. There is pain and stiffness on dorsiflexion and plantar flexion. There is no crepitus.

L5. What is your management plan for this man?

James has a chest x-ray, ECG, troponin level, exercise tolerance test and echocardiogram in the chest pain clinic. Myocardial infarction is excluded as the ECG reveals no abnormality and normal sinus rhythm, and the troponin level was normal. He suffers no chest pain or ECG changes during his exercise tolerance test. Echocardiogram suggests mild left ventricular hypertrophy with a reasonable ejection fraction. There is no significant aortic stenosis or aortic regurgitation. A provisional diagnosis of gastric oesophageal reflux disease is made and he is started on lansoprazole. At a follow up appointment, James says that his chest pain has gone.

The results of his ankle x-ray show moderately severe osteoarthritic changes with osteophytes and narrowing of the joint space. The physiotherapist sees him and treats him initially with ultrasound and teaches him strengthening exercises. On the next visit, the pain is still quite severe so James is given a series of cortisone injections into his left ankle joint. After three months he feels relief from his pain and his walking improves.

Case Study M

Fatima Begum

Fatima, aged 75 years, has suffered from Type 2 diabetes mellitus for the past six years. She takes bendroflumethiazide 2.5 mg daily and amlodipine 10mg daily for hypertension, metformin 500mg three times a day, rosiglitazone 8mg once a day, aspirin 75mg every day, simvastatin 40mg daily, salbutamol 200mcg 2 puffs as required and budesonide metered dose inhaler 200mcg twice daily for asthma prevention.

Today she comes to see you with shortness of breath and fatigue. This came on suddenly three days ago after she had been polishing her furniture. She thought that the spray polish had irritated her chest and brought on an asthma attack. She took her salbutamol inhaler more frequently and has been having 2–4 puffs four hourly, but the breathlessness is still troubling her. She finds she can't lie back in bed as this makes her shortness of breath worse. She has a productive cough with frothy pink sputum.

General survey shows increased respiratory rate and ankle oedema.

M1. What examination and investigations will help you to make a diagnosis?

M2. Explain the provisional diagnosis and differential diagnoses.

Fatima's echocardiogram result shows severe systolic dysfunction and a reduced ejection fraction of 18%. The chest x-ray shows cardiomegaly and the serum brain natriuretic peptide (BNP) levels are raised. This confirms the diagnosis of heart failure.

M3. Describe the pathophysiology of heart failure.

M4. What drug treatment should be initiated for Fatima's left ventricular heart failure?

Case Study N

Mrs Stravinsky

Mrs Stravinsky, aged 82 years, is brought to see you by her daughter-in-law, Teresa. Teresa has come to the UK with her husband to stay with Mrs Stravinsky for a month. She says that her mother-in-law is coughing a lot and appears much thinner than when she last visited one year ago. Mrs Stravinsky lives alone since her husband died ten years ago. Her neighbour gets her shopping for her once a week and collects her repeat prescriptions as she gets too breathless to go out of her flat. She still smokes 5–10 cigarettes every day. She does not drink alcohol. She takes ipratropium bromide 20 mcg/metered inhalation, one to two puffs four times a day via cfc-free inhaler, and salmeterol aerosol inhalation 25mcg/metered inhalation two puffs twice a day. She also takes paracetamol occasionally for osteoarthritis in her knees and lactulose for occasional episodes of constipation. The practice nurse invites Mrs Stravinsky for an annual COPD check up and she attends the surgery using Dial-a-Ride.

Mrs Stravinsky has a hearing aid in her left ear. Despite this, she still has hearing difficulty. She also does not speak much English. With patient questioning of both Mrs Stravinsky and her daughter-in-law, you establish that for the past two months her cough has been more frequent than in the past. She has disturbed nights due to the excessive coughing. The cough is productive and she is bringing up more sputum than usual. Her sputum is usually grey-green in colour, but for the past few weeks it is often 'browny- red'. She has become more tired than usual and regularly has a three-hour sleep after lunch. Teresa says that Mrs Stravinsky has a reasonable appetite and eats three small meals a day and has snacks of tea and biscuits in between meals. Her mother-in-law does not like eating fruit, but has vegetables every day. Her weight today is 48 kilograms. According to her past records her weight two years ago was 56 kilograms.

According to her records, her past medical history includes respiratory infection last year, fracture of the ulna and radius three years ago, knee replacement surgery 15 years ago, diagnosis of COPD 20 years ago and normal vaginal delivery of two children in Poland more than 40 years ago.

You summarise her significant symptoms: increasing cough, increased sputum production, change of colour of sputum from grey-green to browny-red, weight loss, and fatigue.

N1. What are the possible causes for these symptoms?

On examination, there is slight clubbing of the finger nails. She does not have pale conjunctivae suggesting anaemia. There is no evidence of central or peripheral cyanosis. There is no ankle oedema. Her JVP is not raised. There is no lymphadenopathy. There are coarse crackles heard in both lung bases. The respiratory rate is slightly increased at 28 breaths per minute. Her blood pressure is 136/84mmHg, her heart rate is regular, and the first and second heart sound is heard with no added heart sounds or murmurs. Her temperature is normal at 36.5 degrees centigrade.

N2. Explain fine and coarse crackles heard on auscultation.

N3. List five factors that cause increased respiratory rate:

1.

2.

3.

4.

5.

6.

N4. What investigations should be arranged?

Unfortunately chest x-ray shows a shadow in the left lung suggestive of carcinoma. She is referred urgently to the Respiratory Team. Bronchoscopy and biopsy confirm a diagnosis of bronchogenic carcinoma (classified as a non-small-cell lung cancer). CT scans of the brain and bones were negative.

Case Study P

Jerome

Jerome attends the surgery alone saying his carer had told him to attend. The carer has written a note saying that Jerome is unwell with a temperature and is sleeping more than usual. The note also says that he has been ill for ten days. You ask Jerome to tell you about his illness. He says he feels a bit tired, but he has felt tired for a long time since having to take tablets. He shows you his medication card that says Risperidone 6mg daily. According to the electronic medical records, Jerome has been taking Risperidone for four years. On more specific questioning, he denies any pain or loss of appetite. He says he does not smoke cigarettes and you notice that he does not smell of cigarette smoke. He says no when you ask about needing to pass urine more frequently than usual. He says he has not vomited and has no cough.

On examination he appears pale and has a fever of 39.2 degrees centigrade. He is wearing a heavy coat, scarf and hat. His face is flushed and he has beads of sweat on his forehead.

P1. Use your British National Formulary to describe the type of drug that Jerome is taking.

P2. What are the indications for use of this drug?

P3. List the side effects of Risperidone:

P4. Which less common side effect could account for him still wearing winter clothes?

You check his ears with the otoscope. The ear canals and tympanic membranes are normal. You examine his throat and find that his pharynx and tonsils also appear normal. You palpate the lymph nodes of his head and neck and find that he has two slightly enlarged anterior cervical lymph nodes.

P5. List the names of all the lymph nodes found in the head and neck.

You look at Jerome's hands. He has no finger clubbing and no peripheral cyanosis. There are no nicotine stains on his fingers. You then ask him to kindly remove his outdoor clothes and jumper and T-shirt so that you can examine his chest. There is no rash and no scars visible. His respiratory rate is slightly increased at 26 breaths per minute. He has equal lung expansion. You auscultate his lungs and hear crackles in the left lung base. There are no wheezes or rubs. Whilst in the surgery, Jerome coughs frequently and the cough sounds productive. You then ask Jerome if he would manage to pass urine into a pot so that it can be tested for urinary tract infection. He agrees. The urine shows no abnormality on dipstick testing for ketones, nitrate, protein, blood and glucose.

P6. What is your provisional diagnosis?

P7. What do you prescribe?

You make an appointment for Jerome to have a review in three days. He comes in to your room with his carer. The carer says that Jerome's fever has gone and he is much more energetic now. On examination, he still has crackles in his left lung base so you arrange to see him once more in a week's time to confirm that he is making a full recovery.

P8. Jerome attends your surgery for an annual physical health check – what should this include?

Answers

James

L1. Write down six questions you should ask related to his chest pain?

1. Whereabouts in your chest do you feel the pain?
2. Does it come on when you are exerting yourself?
3. Does the pain go away if you rest?
4. Is it worse after a big meal?
5. Is it worse in cold weather?
6. Does the pain come on if you get angry or excited?

L2. Write down three questions you would ask related to his ankle pain:

1. Did the pain in the ankle commence after a recent or long-term injury?
2. Are you still able to walk and go about your usual daily activities?
3. Does the ankle joint sometimes become red and swollen?

L3. Describe your physical examination of the cardiovascular system:

You may only have ten minutes in your consultation, so it may be necessary to carry out a minimal examination of his heart. If time permits you should try to include the following:

Ask for permission to examine James. Take his blood pressure and assess his radial and brachial pulses. Check his face and hands for peripheral cyanosis. Check around his eyes for xanthelasmata and inspect the conjunctivae for anaemia and jaundice. Check his fingernails for clubbing. Then get him to undress to his underpants and lie up on the couch with his upper body at a 45° angle to his legs. Look at his neck to check for raised jugular venous pressure. Inspect his chest for scars, visible heaves or signs of respiratory distress. Palpate the trachea and apex beat to exclude mediastinal shift. Palpate his carotid, femoral, popliteal, posterior tibialis and dorsalis pedis pulses symmetrically. You should note whether all pulses are present or absent and whether pulse volumes are symmetrical. Palpate his anterior chest for heaves which could be a sign of right or left ventricular hypertrophy and thrills which would suggest cardiac murmurs. Auscultate the heart sounds at the aortic, pulmonary, tricuspid and mitral areas, noting the quality of heart sounds one and two (S1 and S2) and listening for third or fourth heart sounds or murmurs. Auscultate the lung bases. Crackles could signify pulmonary oedema secondary to cardiac failure.

L4. Describe your examination of his ankles:

Ask James to remove his trousers, shoes and socks. Ask him to sit up on the couch. Inspect both ankles for deformity, swelling, redness and heat. Compare the painful left ankle with the normal right ankle. Ask James to move his ankles into dorsiflexion, plantar flexion, inversion and eversion of both ankles. Then palpate the ankles for crepitus as you move the ankle. Also inspect the soles of the feet for calluses. Observe for abnormal toe separation or deformity, such as hallux valgus, (bunion) or hammer toe. Gently squeeze the metatarsal head to elicit any tenderness.

L5. What is your management plan for this man?

You should refer James to the chest pain clinic as he has had pain related to exertion for the past two days.

His chest pain may be referred pain from his stomach. Ibuprofen seems to aggravate the pain, so this should be stopped. He should be encouraged to take paracetamol instead, or codeine and paracetamol if the pain is not controlled.

James should also be encouraged to attend the surgery yearly for a hypertension review. This includes checking his lipid profile, blood glucose, renal function and liver function. He should also have his urine dip-stick tested for protein.

You should arrange an x-ray of his left ankle. Regardless of the outcome of the x-ray, James will benefit from physiotherapy for left ankle so this should be arranged. Appropriate analgesia should be prescribed.

Fatima Begum

M1. What examination and investigations will help you to make a diagnosis?

You should check Fatima's blood pressure, respiratory rate, blood glucose and temperature. You should carry out a full cardiovascular and respiratory examination. This includes inspection of the face, hands, neck (JVP) and chest wall. You should palpate the chest wall for respiratory expansion and heaves and thrills, and palpate the pulses. You should percuss the lungs for areas of dullness or hyper-resonance. You should then auscultate the lungs and heart. Patients with heart failure often have a third heart sound. If possible you should check oxygen saturation and brain natriuretic peptide (BNP). You should arrange a chest x-ray. Echocardiogram should also be arranged.

M2. Explain the provisional diagnosis and differential diagnoses.

With the symptoms of orthopneoa, frothy pink sputum and ankle oedema the most likely diagnosis is cardiac failure.

Differential diagnoses could include worsening asthma, chronic obstructive pulmonary disease, chest infection or anxiety.

M3. Describe the pathophysiology of chronic heart failure.

Heart failure is a progressive weakening of the ventricular myocardium which reduces the pumping efficiency of the heart. In a healthy heart there is a balance between cardiac output and venous return. Heart failure leads to an inadequate blood circulation so that the needs of tissues are not met. Damage to the myocardium may be caused by ischaemia due to coronary artery disease. It can also be caused by persistent high blood pressure. When the ventricles are pumping against excessive force in the arteries, the muscles lose their contractility and become permanently stretched. Heart failure can also be the result of mitral or aortic valve disease or cardiomyopathies.

M4. What drug treatment should be initiated for Fatima's left ventricular heart failure?

Treatment is directed at conserving the energy of the heart, reducing blood pressure and removing excess fluid in the body. Fatima already takes amlodipine and bendromethiazide to control her blood pressure. Although she is taking the diuretic bendromethiazide, she has developed pulmonary and ankle oedema, so she would benefit from a loop diuretic.

The National Institute for Clinical Excellence (2003) has produced guidelines for the drug treatment of heart failure due to left ventricular systolic dysfunction. Heart failure is classed as stages 1–4. The guidelines recommend that patients start ACE-inhibitors. Fatima Begum is not currently taking an ACE-inhibitor so this should be started and the dose titrated upwards to the recommended maintenance dose for heart failure.

Mrs Stravinsky

N1. What are the possible causes for these symptoms?

The combination of cough, weight loss and cigarette smoking should alert you to the risk of lung cancer. Alternatively she could have a respiratory infection. Other causes of weight loss in an older person are Type 2 diabetes mellitus, depression, dementia and malnutrition.

N2. Explain fine and coarse lung crackles heard on auscultation.

Fine crackles sound like hairs being rolled together next to your ear. They are usually heard on inspiration. Fine crackles are heard after the small airways close prematurely on expiration as they 'pop' open with the next in-breath.

Coarse crackles are caused by fluid bubbling in the larger airways. They are sometimes reduced or altered if the patient coughs or takes deep breaths.

N3. List five factors that cause increased respiratory rate:

Respiratory rate is increased in lung disease where carbon dioxide is retained. It is common to notice increased respiratory rate in conditions such as:

1. asthma

2. chronic obstructive pulmonary disease

3. pneumothorax

4. pneumonia

5. pulmonary fibrosis

6. pulmonary oedema.

Respiratory rate is also increased in other general conditions such as: fever, acidosis, myocardial infarction, heart failure, anxiety.

Increased respiratory rate is also a normal physiological response to exercise and adjusting to high altitude.

N4. What investigations should be arranged?

Mrs Stravinsky should have a chest x-ray arranged to look for the cause of her worsening respiratory symptoms. Spirometry should be considered if this hasn't been done recently. She should also have the following blood tests arranged to investigate her weight loss: full blood count, random blood glucose, erythrocyte sedimentation rate, thyroid function tests, urea and electrolytes.

Jerome

P1. Use your British National Formulary to describe the type of drug that Jerome is taking?

Risperidone is an atypical antipsychotic medication.

P2. What are the indications for use of this drug?

The indications are acute and chronic psychoses and mania.

P3. List the side effects of Risperidone:

The side effects include: weight gain, dizziness, postural hypotension, extrapyramidal symptoms, hyperglycaemia, insomnia, agitation, anxiety, headache, drowsiness, impaired concentration, fatigue, blurred vision, constipation, nausea and vomiting, dyspepsia, abdominal pain, hyperprolactinaemia, sexual dysfunction, priapism, urinary incontinence, tachycardia, hypertension, oedema, rash, rhinitis, cerebrovascular accident, neutropenia and thrombocytopenia.

P4. Which less common side effect could account for him still wearing winter clothes?

A less common side effect is abnormal temperature regulation. This could explain why Jerome has put on heavy clothes when he has a high temperature and it is not cold outside.

Answers

P5. List the names of the lymph nodes found in the head and neck:

Preauricular, post auricular, occipital, tonsillar, submandibular, submental, anterior cervical chain, posterior cervical chain, supraclavicular.

P6. What is your provisional diagnosis?

Community acquired pneumonia

P7. What do you prescribe?

Amoxicillin 500mg three times a day for ten days (having excluded penicillin allergy)

P8. Jerome attends your surgery for an annual physical health check – what should this include?

Patients who have schizophrenia and take antipsychotic medication have a greater risk of developing diabetes mellitus and ischaemic heart disease. Therefore they should have annual screening of blood pressure, weight, body mass index, waist circumference. Blood tests should be taken for lipids, triglycerides, random blood glucose, urea and electrolytes, liver function tests. Health education should be given regarding smoking cessation, diet and exercise.

Key Texts

Epstein, O., Perkin, G. D., Cookson, J., & de Bono, D. P. (2003). *Clinical Examination*, 3rd Edition. St Louis: Mosby.

Kumar, P. & Clark, M. (2005). *Clinical Medicine*, 6th edn. Edinburgh: W B Saunders.

Marieb, E. & Hoehn, K. (2006). *Human anatomy and physiology*, 7th edn. New Jersey: Pearson International.

National Organisation of Nurse Practitioner Faculties (NONPF) (1995). *Advanced Nursing Practice: Curriculum Guidelines and Program Standards for Nurse Practitioner Education*. Washington: NONPF.

National Organisation of Nurse Practitioner Faculties (NONPF) (2001). *Draft 1: Domains and Competencies of Nurse Practitioner Practice*. September. Washington: NONPF.

Silverman, J., Kurtz, S. & Draper, J. (2005). *Skills for Communicating with Patients*, 2nd edn. London: Radcliffe Press.

Walsh, M. (2005). *Nurse Practitioners: Clinical Skills and Professional Issues*, 2nd edn. Edinburgh: Elsevier Health Sciences.

Further Reading

Hopcroft, K. & Forte, V. (2003). *Symptom sorter*. Abingdon: Radcliffe.

Modell, M., Boyd, R., Mughal, Z. & Mughal M. (1996). *Paediatric Problems in General Practice*, 3rd edn. Oxford: Oxford General Practice.

Stern, S., Cifu, A. & Altkorn, D. (2006). *Symptom to Diagnosis – An Evidence-based Guide*. Berkshire: Lange/McGraw-Hill.

References

Bowling, A. (2005). *Ageing Well – Quality of Life in Old Age*. Berkshire: Open University Press McGraw-Hill Education.

Brindle, P., Emberson, J., Lampe, F., Walker, M., Whincup, P., Fahey, T. & Ebrahim, S. (2003). 'Predictive accuracy of the Framingham Coronary risk score in British men: prospective cohort study' in *British Medical Journal* 327: 1267.

British National Formulary (2007). *British National Formulary 53*. London: BMJ Publishing Group and RPS Publishing.

Centor, R. M., Witherspoon, J. M., Dalton, H. P., Brody, C. E. & Link, K. (1981). 'The diagnosis of strep throat in adults in the emergency room' in *Medical Decision Making* 1: 239–246.

Department of Health (2001). 'Guidance for the field social workers, residential social workers and foster carers providing information and referring young people to contraception and sexual health services.' Available online at www.dh.gov.uk (accessed September 2007).

Department of Health (2004). *The National Health Service Framework for children, young people and maternity services*. London: Department for Education and Skills, Department of Health.

Du Vivier, A. (2002). *Atlas of Clinical Dermatology*, 3rd edn. Oxford: Churchill Livingstone.

Epstein, O., Perkin, G.D., Cookson, J. & de Bono, D. P. (2003). *Clinical Examination*, 3rd edn. St Louis: Mosby

Faculty of Family Planning and Reproductive Health Care Clinical Effectiveness Unit (2003). 'FFPRHC Guidance: first prescription of combined oral contraception' in *Journal of Family Planning and Reproductive Health Care* 29(2), 9–15.

Gonce Morton, P. 1990 *Health Assessment, Nurse's Clinical Guide.* Pennsylvania: Springhouse Corporation.

Haslett, C., Chilvers, E., Boon, N. & Colledge, N. (2002). *Davidson's Principles and Practice of Medicine*. Edinburgh: Churchill Livingstone.

Horrocks, S., Anderson, E. & Salisbury, C. (2002). 'Systematic review of whether nurse practitioners working in primary care can provide equivalent care to doctors' in *British Medical Journal* 324(7341): 819–823.

Illingworth, R. S. (1983). *The Development of the Infant and the Young Child, Normal and Abnormal*. London: Churchill Livingstone.

Jarvis, C. (2004). *Physical Examination and Health Assessment*, 4th edn. St Louis: Saunders.

Johnson, G., Hill-Smith, I. & Ellis, C. (2005). *The Minor Illness Manual*, 3rd edn. Oxford: Radcliffe.

Kurtz, S. & Silverman, J. (1996). 'The Calgary-Cambridge Observation Guides: An aid to defining the curriculum and organising the teaching in communication training programmes' in *Medical Education* 30: 83–89.

Linder, J. A. & Stafford, R. S. (2001). 'Antibiotic treatment of adults with sore throat by Community Primary Care Physicians. A National Survey 1989–1999' in *Journal of the American Medicine Association* 286: 1181–1186.

National Institute for Clinical Excellence (2007). 'Feverish illness in children', Clinical Guideline 47. London: NICE. Available at www.nice.org.uk/CG047

National Institute for Clinical Excellence (2003). 'Management of chronic heart failure in adults in primary and secondary care', Clinical Guideline 5. London: NICE. Available at www.nice.org.uk/guidance/index.jsp?action=byID&o=10924

National Institute for Clinical Excellence (2001). 'Low Back Pain Referral Advice: a guide to appropriate referral from general to specialist services.' London: NICE.

Neighbour, R. (1987). The Inner Consultation. Lancaster: MTO Press.

Nursing and Midwifery Council (2005). 'Implementation of a framework for the standards of post-registration nursing, Agendum 27,1.' Available from https://www.nmc-uk.org/aFreeDisplay.aspx?DocumentID=1669 (accessed September 2007).

Raza, S., Denholm, S. & Wong, J. (1995). 'An audit of the management of acute otitis externa in an ENT casualty clinic' in Journal of Laryngology & Otology 109(2), 130–133.

Royal College of Nursing (2002, revised March 2005). Competencies in Nursing. Nurse Practitioners – an RCN guide to the Nurse Practitioner role, competencies and programme approval. London: Royal College of Nursing.

Royal Pharmaceutical Society of Great Britain (1997). From Compliance to Concordance: Achieving Shared Goals in Medicine Taking. London: Royal Pharmaceutical Society of Great Britain and Merck Sharp and Dohme.

Scottish Intercollegiate Guidelines Network (SIGN) (2003). Diagnosis and management of childhood otitis media in primary care, Report No. 66, Scottish Intercollegiate Guidelines Network.

Silverman, J., Kurtz, S. & Draper, J. (2005). Skills for Communicating with Patients, 2nd edn. London: Radcliffe Press.

Van Zwanenburg, T. & Harrison, J. (2004). Clinical Governance in Primary Care, 2nd edn. Oxford: Radcliffe.

Waddell, G., Feder, G., McIntosh, A., Lewis, M. & Hutchinson, A. (1996). Low Back Pain Evidence Review. London: Royal College of General Practitioners.

Walsh, M. (2005). Nurse Practitioners: Clinical Skills and Professional Issues, 2nd edn. Edinburgh: Elsevier Health Sciences

Weed, L.L. (1969). Medical Records, Medical Education, and Patient Care. The Problem-oriented Record as a Basic Tool. Cleveland, OH: Case Western Reserve University.

Wewers, M. E. & Lowe, N. K. (1990). 'A critical review of visual analogues scales in the measurement of clinical phenomena' in Research in Nursing and Health 13, 227–236.

www.backcare.org.uk (accessed June 2007).
www.cks.library.nhs.uk/Acne_vulgaris/In_depth/References (accessed May 2007).
www.cks.library.nhs.uk/back_pain_lower (accessed August 2007).
www.cks.library.nhs.uk/eczema_atopic
www.cks.library.nhs.uk/otitis_externa (accessed October 2007).
www.cks.library.nhs.uk/patient_information_leaflet/corticosteroid_preparations_topical
www.cks.library.nhs.uk/patient_information_leaflet/emollients/introduction
www.cks.library.nhs.uk/Pyelonephritis_acute (accessed July 2007).
www.cks.library.nhs.uk/search/0/urinary_tract_infection (accessed July 2007).
www.depression-primarycare.co.uk/images/PHQ-9.pdf (accessed October 2007).
www.earcarecentre.com (accessed October 2007).
www.entnursing.com (accessed October 2007).
www.jointzone.org.uk (accessed July 2007).
www.patient.co.uk/showdoc/23068674/
www.patient.co.uk/showdoc/23068864/
www.patient.co.uk/showdoc/23068975/
www.perthes.org.uk (accessed June 2007).